THE
HUMAN DIET

COPYRIGHT: Richard H. Hendry,
2018/2023

THE HUMAN DIET

HENDRY'S 3 LAWS FOR HUMANS:

1) Never accept any argument that is made in favor for a chemical and against nature

2) Never accept trading moments of bliss for years of pain

3) Protect your body and your world – you only get one.

THE HUMAN DIET

This book is not intended as a substitute for the medical advice of physicians. The reader should regularly consult a physician in matters relating to his/her health and particularly with respect to any symptoms that may require diagnosis or medical attention.

THE HUMAN DIET

Forward

Talk about food

I do a lot of talking about food.
You hear a lot about food.
Everybody you know has their own take
on what food you should eat.

From the veg heads to Paleo to the Atkins
mad pork rind eater and everywhere in
between.
On the one hand you've got the AMA's
that cling to the titanic bound food
pyramid.
Then you've got the veg-heads that
proclaim that we have a GI track like a
monkey- therefore we must eat like a
monkey.
The latest findings from the human
genome project says we are real close to
pigs...yes, pigs.
And if that is not enough we've got diets
from all over the world, macrobiotic from
Asia.
The Dosha diets from India. The diet
Mediterranean from, well you know... the
Mediterranean.

Then we've got the blood type diet, the body ecology diet, the zone diet, the protein power diet, the carbo addicts diet, caveman diets and my favorite the cabbage soup diet.

And intermittent Fasting aka – I forget to eat, so now that is intention!

Also, everywhere you look there's a diet or diet product vying for you belief and cash. The Metabo-lifers, the carbo blocker, fat blocker, caffeine raging, ma hung, ginseng, themogenic fuel to burn you brown fatty tissue to death.

The M-deities are not far behind, with a little help from Phizer and other drug companies ran by the dark lord himself.

They have real bad stuff like Phen Phen and Meridian all designed to kill you by stopping your body from asking for food! do you see point here; it's if you're dead... your weight is not an issues.

Sometimes I get going on a rant. Sorry, it's just that all of this is stupid.
That's right, stupid. And all of these things are designed to fool or trick your body into doing something rather then feeding it right and making it healthy.

In all of these attempts at murder, no one ever says anything about your diet...

Wait....I know what you're going to say.
I've read this book too.
They talk a lot about "A Diet" that you should follow and why....but they never talk about YOU.
Well you might say that's splitting hairs, it is not - they do not know you.
So why do you think that someone that has never met you and knows nothing about you can give you a diet that will work?

There is only one you.
And how you metabolize, digest, absorb, utilize and eliminate is all you!

Now hold on... the ride gets rough from here on out.
I lose most of the people I talk too right here. Most think "if I cannot listen to these others, why should I listen to you?'.

That's a fair question; the reason is that I am not going to give you a diet idea that works on some people to lose weight.

I am not going to say take this and you will lose weight and if it does not work... take more.

Some people think that I mean that you must have a bunch of tests and get a diet from that.
NO, the truth is that a little common sense and understanding of your body, lifestyle and environmental factors will give you the diet, supplements and other factors you need to live a health life.
It lacks the glamour of that magic pill or the fun of the all peanut butter diet, but trust me... being health is worth the effort.

The problem is that almost everyone I see says the same thing

"Everyone I talk to tells me something different".

I get this one a lot.
Most of you have come to the healthy conclusion that we do not know what we're talking about.
And why not?, if you took your car to 10 shops and every one told you the other guy were wrong, you'd be stumped.

Or might you do what I did, I bought the book on my car and studied it.
 I got tired of thinking that every time I took my car to the shop, I was charged 100.00 for a 5.00 part or a loose wire.

I am not suggesting that you go to school
for years to understand your body...if you
decide to do that, I'd be happy to have
you out here with me.
But it is not really necessary.

What then will I tell you that none of these
other books have not?

The truth about our diet today and
yesterday. The truth about your body,
what it's made of and what we have in
common.

The truth about the world we live in and
why we are in the shape we're in.

Most importantly is that you must do this.
Only you can help you, not me. I can only
help you to understand that you have
been told nothing about how things really
work.

Those sound bites about the benefits of
vitamin C or Phyto Estrogens are just
parts of the big puzzle that is your health.

The main reason I call this book – the
human diet, is that almost no one wants
to talk about the elephant in the room.
You are human – a natural occurring life
form on this planet.

And as such, there is a human diet that should be the base foods you eat.
The problem is that you have no earthly idea what it is and what it is not.

Its not your fault, you've been lied to since the day you were born.

It has not been an international conspiracy (or has it? Just kidding) it has been a convergence of bad ideas, misconceptions, convenience and necessity for survival.

Lets take these on one by one and they are easy to find – they all converge in the one place – the pyramid.

CHAPTER ONE

Thriving vs. Surviving

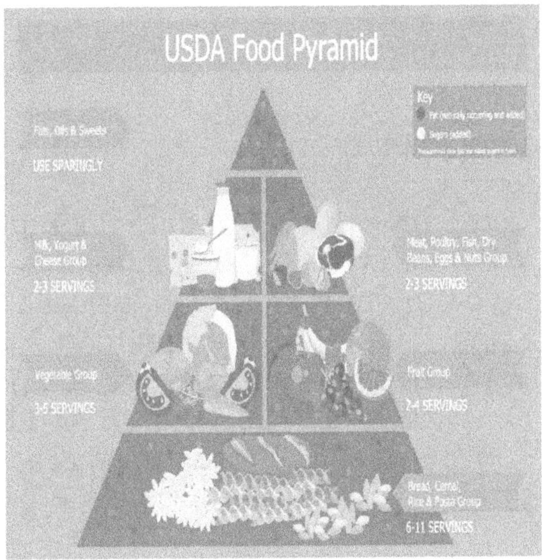

Take this work of art, the long covenanted
and insidious lie of the food pyramid.
This is not science – it does not, in any
way, represent what a human needs.

It is a construct of the foods available in the country. And while that fact is well known (or should be by this point) we still see this thing everywhere.

When people ask me about a pyramid, I tell them they were tombs!!!!!
This little disaster is responsible for more deaths and suffering than the last 5 wars!

Harsh?
Yes.
But none the less true.

They keep reworking it and up dating it, this one here is the 2018 update but it still asked you to eat more bread, grains, pasta and cereal then the real food.
 When there is no evidence that you need ANY OF THOSE THINGS TO LIVE AT ALL!
And – in truth, all of those things are man- made.

6-11 servings of things that need to be processed in order for you to digest them.

How could that be right?
How could that be a natural diet?
We are the only inhabitants of this planet that eat, almost exclusively, foods that are not found in nature in there original form.

GRAINS

Grains historically, need to be cracked, soaked or fermented in order to be consumed.
Cows do this in their multi stomach system – in ever sense, this food is not human food....it is our food's food! And even our food's food should not be grain...they really only need grass to get everything they need.

Grass is what all grain start out as and if it were being eaten by the cows they would be healthier and healthier for us.

Grain (post grass) does only one thing – makes you and your food – FAT.
If that were not enough, today we do even more to grains in order to make the process quicker. Taking more out of grains then ever before and leaving you and your food nothing.
So why do we cling to it so tightly?
The answer is simple – grain, like a number of things we eat, are foods of necessity.

The very latest guess on how long humans have been eating grain is now around 100,000 years.
And to some that makes it OK.

In fact, they have found tools used for grinding grains back as far as 105,000 years. Again this is now used to argue that it has been part of the human diet so long that somehow that makes it good for us. The problem with this is that it was still being processed.

Wither its in a factory today or on a stone 100,000 years ago – we still had to process it!
Yes we used it to get by, yes it kept the race alive and yes you can get by on it today. The issue is not just about getting by on it – its about thriving – not merely surviving. Its not an original human food, just one of many we used to get by on.

We could also make a point of saying that these grains 100,000 years ago were not sprayed with presides or chemically fertilized.
That they contained way more nutrient then the grains today.
 And that while they were used – they in no way comprised 55% of the human diet but that's all just window dressing.

End of the day – its just not human food.
They are still being pushed due to the fact
that we have gone to trouble of growing
them everywhere and basing a huge part
of commerce on them.
They can be made into all sorts of yummy
stuff and hold longer than meats which is
why they ended up as a staple of our diet
back when we had little in the way of
preserving foods.
Sure they will make you move your bowels
but so will greens – so why would we
choose the empty grain for that one
reason?
When we could use the greens and also
get all the nutrient? I
ts a hollow argument.
Think of it as money.
Imagine there are two envelopes on the
table -both 3 inches thick. One is filled
with one dollar bills and the other is filled
with 100 dollar bills.
If I offered you either -which one would
you choose?
When we think of it that way -the choice is
simple.
The problem is that we do not think about
it.
Instead we let other non- nutrient factors
cloud the decision.

Non- Nutrient Factors:
these are things we consider that are not related in any way to whats best for us. They include; taste, color, texture, packaging, shape, experience and recognition.

Absurd right?
I mean if someone told you they took the one dollar bills because they like the design of it more than the hundreds – you might try to get them Baker acted!

When you separate the bull from the fact – there is no good argument for grains.

So we have to amputate the bottom of the pyramid.

As a side note on the ancient grain issue – you should know that the Egyptians from 3000 years ago had a lot of the so called "modern diseases" as did many other very old cultures.
 Using CT scans – researchers in 2014 scanned 76 mummies from Egypt that were 3000 years old. They also scanned 61 Peruvians ranging from 600 to 2000 years old along with Native Americans from 1600 years ago.

They found that they had all the markers of heat diseases, clogged arteries and were at risk of strokes. And they all ate diets that are suggested today to help reduce heart disease!

Going back further, Dr. Barry Sears (author of The Zone books) noted that when grains were first introduced into the human diet, three things immediately happened:
1) Mankind shrunk in size from lack of adequate protein.
2) Diseases of "modern civilization," such as heart attacks and arthritis, first appeared.
3) Obesity became prevalent.
How do we know these things?
From studies of Egyptian mummies.

Not only were Egyptians much shorter than neo-paleolithic man, but they also showed significant indications of heart disease.
Furthermore, Egyptians had the same amount of obesity as found in the U.S. today.
We can determine this from the excess amount of skin found around the stomachs of preserved mummies.
And grain and soil content have not improved with the centuries.

  Lastly, when someone tells you about our lifespans and that we live longer now than before. You will need to apply some facts to that statement.
One of the most repeated half truths is that our modern diet is responsible for longer life.
It is not.
Its a great sound bite. It gives us a big pat on the back. It is just not, what you would call, true.

The truth is that mortality rates of the young were reduced. 0 – 5 death rates before the industrialized world were super high. Being able to save the live of newborns and keep children alive beyond 5 and then beyond 12 – skewed these numbers.
When you look at 12 – death number – we have not increased life spans in over 2,000 years.
The other factors were advancements in medication and procedures. And elder health. Simply being able to keep older people alive longer through nursing and continued care.
However, when you look at these factors, it is about fixing broken stuff.

Not prevention through good nutrition.

And absent of these medical
advancements.

We would still be dying at the same rates.

It is not a good endorsement for the diets
we have been eating since the agricultural
revolution.

THE HUMAN DIET

MILK

Our next big food of survival is dairy. It is in the same class of bad ideas as grains. Only this is our food's babie's food!!
Notice a pattern here?

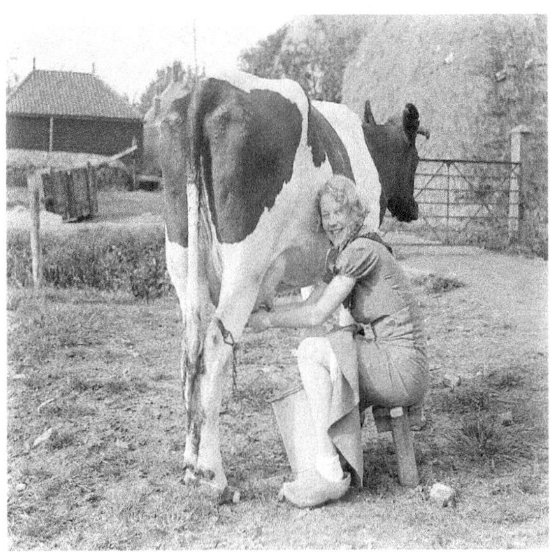

We eat cows, so whatever a cow eats – we should eat?

How did this start?

The best guess on the history of cows'
milk is around 10,000 BCE.

Nomadic tribes stopped moving and
settled down in farming communities.
This era is known as the agricultural
revolution, and with it came domesticated
animals and the advent of by-products
such as milk.

Later, in ancient Egypt, milk and other
dairy products were available, but
reserved for royalty, priests and the very
wealthy.
Around the 5th century AD in western
Europe milk was taken from both cows
and sheep and by the 14th century, cows'
milk was more popular.

While some place the consumption of milk
back even further in history – it all
revolves around this agricultural upstart.

That sounds good in one respect but, if
you were to describe that time as the time
we started to change the way things
worked and the way stuff grew – it starts
to sound like us screwing with nature.

We got tried of chasing our food as it
naturally migrated and found some way to
stay put in a safe climate and survive.

The natural way of doing things was abandoned and the trade off was that we lost foods to thrive on and got foods to survive on.
This was also the case in areas of the world where there were less grazing land.

We penned the animals and used the by-products for survival. It took far less time and effort to drink milk (which was made everyday by cows) then to kill and render an animal.
Plus the meat would not keep long but the milk flowed all the time due to our constant milking.
This dairy thing is the very best example of a food of necessity.
Later, in the late 1800's we started to play with milk to make it safer. Commercial pasteurization was introduced in 1885 and shortly after, milk made the quantum leap from a farm food to widespread consumption.
Sure it lasted longer but, it was more than 80% dead! Save for some fats, protein and a sugar (lactose) that we have a really hard time breaking down.
This change places it on the table of the bulk of humans just a little over a hundred years ago! This is a very new food... driven by commerce, not found in nature for us to consume.

Its all about commerce.

A milk cow is far more valuable than a meat cow.
And we have gotten really good at exploiting them.
Before, we just kept milking them and they kept lactating.
Today high powered machines suck them dry for years.
Check off dairy as a survival food and cut out another section of the evil pyramid.

VEGETABLES
With those two section of pyramid gone,
one would think that what remains sounds
like good advice.
The truth is harder to deal with. If you
look closely at the vegetable section of the
chart – there is something else very
wrong.
Lets start with things like roots.
These would be your potatoes, carrots,
sweet potatoes, onions etc..

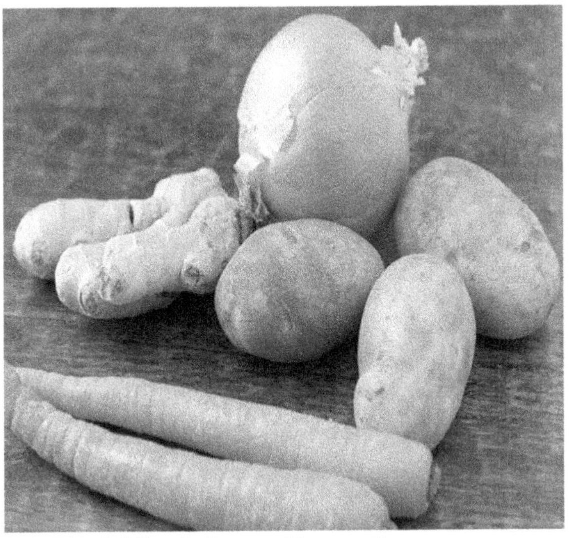

Why would I pick on these?

Let me count the ways.

1. Because you are a human and you do not have a snout. You do not root of food in the ground.

2. It is ecologically unsound to eat the root of a plant. Eat the root – kill the plant.

3. These type of so called vegetables contain more starch and sugar then most above ground vegetables. They effect human blood sugar level wildly and can increase body fat and imbalance human hormones.

4. Most of them have to be cooked to be consumed by humans - so we need that processing again which is a dead give-a-way that its not human food.

5. In general, the green leafy part of any plant or vegetable has way more nutrient in it than the roots.

In fact -
A new analysis published in the journal Hort Science, found the leaves of sweet potatoes have 3 times more vitamin B6, 5 times more vitamin C, and almost 10 times more riboflavin than actual sweet potatoes.

Nutritionally, this makes the greens similar to spinach, but sweet potato leaves have less oxalic acid, which gives some greens like spinach and chard a sharper taste.

The tops of roots mostly can not be eaten raw and some are deadly to humans.

This really puts them in a section of "leave them for the pigs" and to scrub the air!
Placing these that these roots as a food of survival.

Plus the amount of area and time used in planting and replanting these roots is huge and costly.

And again – we are eating the animal's food!!! so even when they think they are right – they still are wrong.

Next on the vegetable section that should not be there is tomatoes – which is a fruit!

Now I know its splitting hairs but if your going to recommend things – you should be accurate about them.
Tomatoes do meet the human food standard because they are above ground, pick-able and eatable raw.

How much of them we should eat is a point of interest as far as the true human diet.
Because of their short season and ripeness issues and geography – tomatoes should be eaten in season like fruit (cause it is one) or for our proposes – in rotation.

 Not a full time food of consumption.

In short – green vegetables that are pick-able and above ground are best and the healthiest for the human.

FRUIT

Skipping over to the right in the now almost deconstructed pyramid to the fruit section – (where the tomato belongs, just saying) we find a lot of great fruit loaded with nutrient.

The one exception is the banana, which is technically a fruit because it contains seeds but its from a herb bush, not a tree.

And since commercially grown bananas are sterile – the banana is in a class all by itself.

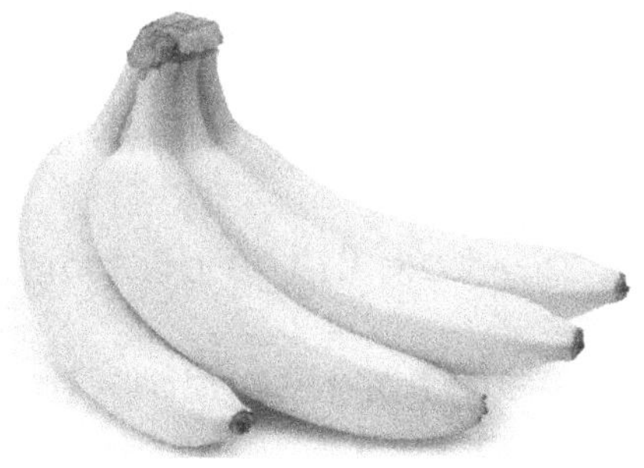

We started eating bananas about 5000 BCE to 8000 BCE in southeast Asia.

Its only due to transplanting, worldwide cultivation over 4000 years and now crop rotation and transportation that you can get a banana in Maine in winter!

Which is to say that not all fruits are equal when it comes to the human diet.

The banana are also very high in sugar on the glycemic chart. As a recommendation - this fruit/herb has more than its share of problems.

You'll find that tropical sourced fruits are best kept in the "every once in a while" column.

In general all fruit should be consumed in small doses. Their short window of ripeness, varied locations and high sugar content makes them lowest on the list of daily foods.

Oops, another hole in the pyramid.

And now for the hardest part – the very top of the stack – at number one on the least loved, most talked about and completely misunderstood macro nutrient – FAT

FATS

With all my heart, I wish that someone, somewhere would have named these things something other than "fat". I'm not kidding here, it would have saved us a lot of trouble.

The word "fat" has such emotion attached to it that its hard to break people from their hate on these poor little life giving and life saving lipids. These little guys and girls are such an important part of our human suit yet at every turn – war is waged on them.

Fat has been on the receiving end of the most ill advised and ill researched attack in human history. We have a Pavlovian recoil when the word is uttered.

A learned response that causes us to want to run and hide and find a mirror quickly in order to see if we have any of it hanging out or off of us in view of the public.

Hundreds of billions of dollars have been spent on weight loss and fat research.
And still the average person has no idea whats good for them.

How we got to the place where one of the three most important things for our life was all but removed from the our diets is the fault of one guy!!!

one F#$king guy!!!!!

In the foul year of our lord - 1958, an American scientist named Ancel Keys started a study called the Seven Countries Study.
He examined the association between diet and cardiovascular disease in different countries.
The study revealed that the countries where fat consumption was the highest had the most heart disease, supporting the idea that dietary fat caused heart disease.
The problem is that he intentionally left out:
1. Countries where people eat a lot of fat but have little heart disease, such as Holland and Norway.
2. Countries where fat consumption is low but the rate of heart disease is high, such as Chile.

3. Well known cultures around the world that had high animal fat consumption and long healthy lives.

Basically, he only used data from the countries that supported his theory, a process known as cherry picking or conformation bias.

This flawed observational study gained massive media attention. And had a major influence on the dietary guidelines of the next few decades.
What followed was the most unexpected turn of events.
In 1977, an American committee of the U.S. senate led by George McGovern published the first Dietary Goals For The United States in order to reverse the epidemic of heart disease in the country.

The recommend diet was based on Keys work, work the experts in the health field at the time knew were wrong.
These guidelines received major criticism at the time from many respected scientists like John Yudkin
(who rightly insisted that sugar was to blame)
and even the American Medical Association!

Basically, the dietary goals were:
1 Eat less fat and cholesterol.
2 Less refined and processed sugars.
3 More complex carbohydrates from
          vegetables, fruits and grains.

These guidelines were picked up by the USDA.
Basically, a low-fat, high-carb diet for everyone. The whole guidelines were based on observational studies made by biased scientists and had nothing even closely resembling scientific proof to back them up.

Since then, many randomized controlled trials have shown that this dietary approach doesn't really work for the people it was meant to help.

What came next, you ask?
An interesting fact - the obesity epidemic started around the time these guidelines were published and the type 2 diabetes epidemic followed soon after. This nonsense had a multi effect on the general public;
1. They were told to randomly remove fat without replacing it with any good fat. In that environment – all fat was bad.

2. By telling people to abstractly reduce fat – they removed meat from the diet in a way that was unexpected and very damaging.
3. The demand for low fat foods and products caused a flood of new and even worse fat substitutes to arrive on the market.
From a sharp increase in fake butter products to other ill advised choices.

This was compounded by Ancel's claims that vegetable oils had a benefit – people started to consume vegetable oils at a wild level.
An oil that for the most part – we had never in taken before and that was not part of a real human diet.
Oils that when heated for cooking, baking or frying became loaded with free radicals and are actually damaging for the heart and arteries and is clinically linked to cancers.

4. All the investment in these "fat free" or "low fat" products and the marketing behind them flooded the airwaves, billboards and TV until everyone just bought in. No one ever bothered to question that the rate of heart disease was still going up.

And when people did – the standard answer was that the public was not following the governments advise.
Mind you – these products filled the shelves!
Which is ridiculous because if no one was buying them they would go out of business.
Instead – you can still find them on the shelves today
It was a perfect storm; marketing, money and mayhem for the 25 years that followed.
The results of this countrywide mass study was alarming – we were fatter, sicker and more confused then ever.

All the favorite diseases that we had been trying to get ride of were up - plus cancer and type II diabetes was raising at a freighting rate.

One of the most shameful results was childhood obesity – 4 generations of children massively overweight and a rise in childhood disease.

This was a dark chapter in our history. Bringing the richest country in the world to a triple epidemic of malnutrition, obesity and disease.

While leaving the public stunned and incapable of believing any advice.
To this day, people still have a hangover of fear about fats and little understanding why we need them.
Here is a small list of the benefits from healthy, natural dietary fat;

A source of energy – Our body uses the fat we eat, and fats we make from other nutrients in our bodies, to provide the energy for most of our life-functions

Energy store – The extra calories that we consume, but do not need to use immediately, are stored for future use in special fat cells (adipose tissue)

Essential fatty acids – Dietary fats that are essential for growth development and cell functions, but cannot be made by our body's processes

Proper functioning of nerves and brain- fats are part of myelin- a fatty material which wraps around our nerve cells so that they can send electrical messages. Our brains contain large amounts of essential fats

Maintaining healthy skin and other tissues. All our body cells need to contain some fats as essential parts of cell membranes, controlling what goes in and out of our cells

Transporting fat-soluble vitamins A, D, E and K through the bloodstream to where they are needed

And the hardest part to believe is that we specifically need cholesterol in the body, yep....we need it!

Here's a few reasons why:

Vitamin D
Cholesterol is a precursor to one of the most important vitamins, vitamin D. Manufacture of vitamin D occurs in the skin, triggered by exposure to sunlight. The ultraviolet B rays in sunlight act as a co-factor for vitamin D production, which requires cholesterol as a starting material. Although fortified foods and some animal foods such as meat and eggs provide small amounts of vitamin D, your body depends significantly on its own ability to produce this important vitamin from cholesterol.

Steroid Hormones

Cholesterol is the basic building block of all steroid hormones.

These include the sex hormones, testosterone, made mainly in the testes in men, and estrogen and progesterone, made mainly in the ovaries in women.

Men's bodies make some estrogen and progesterone. Women's bodies make some testosterone but in much smaller quantities.

Cortisol and asteroidal are also steroid hormones, produced in the adrenal gland and crucial for regulation of blood pressure, responding to stress, maintenance of salt and water balance and proper function of your immune system. For each hormone, cholesterol is modified in a specific way by cells of these organs.

Bile Acids

Bile acids are specialized compounds manufactured in the liver from cholesterol. They are very important in allowing your digestive system to break down fats.

When you eat, bile acids are released into the intestines as part of bile.

These molecules have special characteristics that allow them to form a bridge between fat molecules and water. This emulsifies the fat, making it soluble in the intestinal fluid where enzymes are able to break it down.

So what a great idea it was to just cut it all out and tell people it was death!

Causing damage in a whole host of ways and never effecting any change in the rates of the targeted diseases.

While also allowing manufactured fake substances to further damage us in new and different way.
Talk about a lose – lose!

The best types of fat are the ones found in nature. Animal fats, nut and fruit oils like avocados and coconut. These are not to be avoided and should be used first before anything else.
They make food taste good and feed your body and brain. The plus of good fat consumption is it stops us from craving and we get more energy from fat then any other macro nutrient. And for more recent epidemics of Alzheimer and ADD and Autism these fats are so important that it can not be overstated.

There is new research that is linking these disease's to a lack of good fats.

We should be getting a healthy amount of these fats each day.

Eat fat – do not be afraid.

Like everything else, we want to eat the substance in its most natural form and with as little processing as possible.

The fat contained in natural human foods are made for us to eat and break down and use for body repair and functions. Adding non-food content fat or deep frying in fat is not a healthy choice.

Now with the food pyramid completely torn down, we can start to build a better diet – one is closer to the human diet.

But before you run out to your local grocery – be warned... You may not find what your looking for there.

So first – take a little trip with me to the store.

You might see it very differently now – but there's more work to be done here.

Chapter 2

There is no Twinkie tree

That's right, the Twinkie is not found in nature.
Nor is its natural predator, the cup cake.
Never will you see herds of wild tofu taking to hoof on the open plains.

Also, after much ado it turns out there is no juice or tea or coffee underground springs.
The pasta plant is only a fairy tale that Tony Saprano use to tell Meadow when she was a little girl.
You're wondering what I'm talking about?
Our trip to the food store has uncovered strange things.
Cardboard boxes, metal cans and plastic bags filled with items not found in nature.
And it's not just snack cakes and candy, but things like vegetable trapped in tin cans or imprisoned in frozen tombs.
Refined gains molded into strange designs and patterns. Fruit, ripped open and their insides pressed out into clear glass containers.
Cover the children's eyes, it's horrifying.
What has happened to the food?

Stranger yet is the whole meals in boxes that are not refrigerated.

Over in the meat department, the meats all have a label saying that a 12% solution has been added and the Radura sign lets us know that we are safe from bacteria by the benefits of nuclear radiation.

Over in the produce department, things seem normal, but under closer inspection, we find that the tomatoes have fish enzymes and antibiotic genes.

The vegetables have a high gloss shine from wax, and most everything you taste has the
"Less flavor, looks great" to it.

Hold on to the kids tightly, don't let them wonder...we are about to enter the dairy department.
We do not want to use it anyhow but - All the milk is dead.

 Any benefits that might be drawn from the cow juice have been left on the editing floor at Pasture's lab of,

"Kill them all, let God sort them out."

The cheese is now called cheese food,
why?
Because it is not real cheese.

The stuff still being called cheese is all low
fat...from that low fat cow. The colors are
pretty and the shelf life is long.

Later on our trip we encounter the impulse
racks by the checkout lines and the
manger tells us that of the top 10 items
people buy at the food store are;
Soda
Beer
Smokes of different kinds fill out the top 8
with white bread
Kraft Mac & cheese (food) coming in at 9
and 10.

We leave the store confused, sickened and
still look for FOOD.

Now I know that was a little over the top,
but none the less true.
Where is the food?

The hardest thing for people to get is that
85% of what we eat is not natural – and in
truth – a lot of it isn't even food!

All the stuff in your house that comes in
boxes, tin cans or plastic bags should go.

Lets get to the part where we put the new diet together.
First, we are going to need a set of rules.

CHAPTER 3
RULES AND RATIOS

1st. Rule of shopping
Buy nothing from the inside aisles of the store.

This is true even if you shop at the health food store, although the boxed goodies are made from natural ingredients, they are not found in that form in nature. Your time spent at the grocery store will be cut in half.

All the real food (for the most part) can be found on the walls of the store. Produce, Meat & Seafood, Eggs, butter etc.

Now you will have to wander into the forbidden zone for your Olive oil and tomato sauce (unless you make the sauce yourself?...too much to ask?, ok let's keep going)

Also, herbs and salad dressings will asked you to find them on an inside lane. Other than those exceptions, you'll be making a circle and heading for the check out.

Most asked question is...

So, what should I eat?

If we were to eat a diet of naturally occurring foods, as nature intended. It can be best summed up like this:

Pick it off a plant or tree and hunt, kill it!

Even without the simplest of processes-heat, you could eat these things.
Everything else is changed some way by man.
As you know man does not have a good track record of making things better.

A simple qualifying question to ask is:

Can this be eaten raw?

So what can you eat raw?
Nuts - Seeds
Vegetables – Fruit (in season)
Eggs - Beef – Fish
note; (You cannot eat raw chicken or raw pork, so those are not human food.)

Road block
"You can't eat raw meat; therefore we should not eat meat"

We can eat raw meat.

We have chosen not to for many years.

Now I'm not telling you to eat raw meat.

Its just part of the "rule process" for you to judge what is real human food.

The French eat steak Tar Tar all the time.

In Africa, not only do many tribes still eat raw meat but a few get all their protein from drinking ox blood.

Just because we do not eat it today, does not mean it is not part of our original diet.

I'm saying that it is possible and therefor it must be human food.

Also, it does not mean that we should not incorporate it into our diet.
Should you eat nothing but meat?...NO.
Should you eat no meat? NO.

With that settled let take a look at some of the best protein for humans and why they are so good.

THE EGG

1. Eggs, soft boiled, up or over light.

No scrambled eggs or hard boiled eggs.
Solidifying the yoke or blending them and
exposing them to heat - reduces the
benefit of the lipids – keep them as close
to raw as possible.

Eggs also have the highest uptake of
nitrogen of any human protein source
(which means less nitrogen waste to
protect your bones and other uses of
calcium)
….Eggs are good for you.

They are possibly the best proteins on the
planet.
Egg do not increase cholesterol – if this
comes as a shock to you it would not
surprising.
Egg have been beaten (pardon the pun)
for over 50 years now and little truth has
found it's way into the main stream.
So, how did all this start?

A little history on the flawed study of eggs
and cholesterol:

1) 1979 - Rhesus <u>monkeys</u> fed a diet rich in egg yolks that developed hypercholesterolemia, xanthomatosis and atherosclerosis.

2) In 1908, Ignatowski showed that meat – containing the pro-oxidant iron – fed to <u>adult rabbits</u>, or milk and egg yolks fed to weanling rabbits, induced atherosclerosis.

3) In 1913, Anitschkov established the cholesterol-fed <u>rabbit</u> as a model for dietary atherosclerosis. Cholesterol feeding in rabbits not only causes cholesterol accumulation in plasma and the arterial wall.

On the surface these studies may be taken to be solid. The problem with them is not readily obvious to the average person. On closer inspection, we can see one very big problem;

Every one of the test subjects are naturally herbivores! Yep, they used test subjects that never eat meat or eggs!!!!! Their bodies and its systems are not designed to consume or break down animal fats!!!

The main issue with these tests is that the researchers started off with the idea that humans are vegetarians!
It was, at best, flawed research and at worst – dangerous (at least to the rabbits and monkeys). And in the end showed nothing about how humans use and absorb fats. And again, the increase in those diseases continued in the face of reducing fats.

We started to replace these natural fats with fake products that really do damage the body and hurt the heart.

Lastly, the most recent of these flawed tests was 1979!!! almost 40 years ago. Hardly relevant to you today.

Since these foolish tests where done, science had charged forward and today we have hard evidence that eating eggs does not increase serum cholesterol levels.

A new study from the University of Eastern Finland shows that a relatively high intake of dietary cholesterol, or eating one egg every day, are not associated with an elevated risk of incident coronary heart disease.

Furthermore, no association was found among those with the APOE4 phenotype, which affects cholesterol metabolism and is common among the Finnish population.

The findings were published in the American Journal of Clinical Nutrition in 2016.

The study found that a high intake of dietary cholesterol was not associated with the risk of incident coronary heart disease -- not in the entire study population nor in those with the APOE4 phenotype.

Moreover, the consumption of eggs, which are a significant source of dietary cholesterol, was not associated with the risk of incident coronary heart disease.

The study did not establish a link between dietary cholesterol or eating eggs with thickening of the common carotid artery walls, either.

So, why do you not know this already?

Walking back a half century of mistakes and poorly researched advice is not easy to do and those that have been wrong are not motivated to set the record right.

On top of this – the fat free, low cholesterol food business is huge.

As is the egg replacement industry – AKA - breakfast cereal!

Of course we should be eating natural, cage free, free range eggs and only having them – like all foods – in moderation. But...eat the egg!

FISH

Fish, fresh water and salt water.

The kind a human could catch.

Salmon – wild caught not farmed is the best of all. Followed by Tuna.
These fish have the 2nd highest uptake of nitrogen after eggs.
The healthy fats in fish help with brain function, hormone production and a host of other things in the body.

Although not as high in healthy omega-3 fatty acids as some saltwater fish, freshwater fish are a nutritious choice.

Most freshwater fish are low in fat and high in protein. One serving of most freshwater fish provides more than 30 percent of the dietary reference intake of protein for adults.

Wild Alaskan salmon is the healthiest salmon.

The regulated safe fishing practices used to capture the salmon and the wild, natural diet they consume render it healthy for the palate and the environment.

The calorie and fat content in wild salmon is lower compared with farmed salmon.

Tuna The health benefits of tuna fish include its ability to reduce cardiovascular conditions.
Stimulate growth and development, lower blood pressure and cholesterol levels.
Aid in weight loss efforts, boost the immune system.
Increase energy, maintain the health of the skin, increase red blood cell count, prevent cancer, protect against various kidney diseases.
Reduce general inflammation, and inhibit cell membrane damage.

Other fresh water fish:
Bass
Perch
Walleye and trout are low in calories and high in protein, beneficial oils and low in bad fats.

A FEW FISHY ISSUES

The 2 big issue now days revolves around fish farms and toxicity of saltwater fish.

The first one is easy – NO farm fish.

They do not eat a naturally occurring diet and are in a close environment that is over crowded. Fresh caught and wild is still the best and you should demand it.

This will take you to seafood shops rather then your normal grocery store but its worth it.

The mercury and other contaminants is an other thing all together and here's why:

Mercury is a neurotoxin that affects the brain and nervous system and is particularly dangerous for women who are pregnant as it can have adverse effects on a child's development. Once released into the environment, inorganic mercury is converted to organic mercury (methylmercury) which is the primary form that accumulates in fish and shellfish.

Tile fish usually have the highest levels measuring as many as 1.45 parts per million of mercury.

Other fish found to have high levels of mercury include grouper, swordfish, Spanish mackerel, Chilean sea bass, yellow fin tuna and canned albacore tuna.

Species such as cod, halibut, lobster, snapper and canned tuna contain moderate amounts of mercury. Other fish meeting the threshold of more than 0.5 parts per million of mercury, include king mackerel, shark, marlin, orange roughy and both bigeye and ahi tuna.

Because mercury levels build up in the blood over time, it is best to eat other large fish with high levels of mercury sparingly.
Eating three servings or less of these fish per month prevents side effects from mercury.
Fish with the lowest mercury levels include smaller species of both fish and shellfish.
These varieties include anchovies, crabs, salmon and sardines catfish, clams, scallops and tilapia have the least amounts of mercury.

Freshwater trout, shrimp, oysters and flounder are other safe choices. People can eat these as often as desired unless local advisories warn of higher-than-normal mercury levels.

BEEF

Beef, grass fed, organic beef that is fed no corn or grain has the same healthy fats as fish!

Keep it fresh, not frozen.

Never overcook it and no ground beef! Just good old fashion steaks and roasts.

Beef is good for you, while the bulk of what you have been told about beef is rotates around it being an empty heart attacking product – the true is that beef is high in many things we need to build cells and function.

Beef has one of the highest net uptakes of nitrogen (after eggs and fish) which we need to make every cell in the body.

A quick look at whats in it will make you wonder why we ever stopped eating it.

L-Carnitine

Why is L-Carnitine Important?
Among other functions, L-carnitine plays a part in fat metabolism. L-Carnitine does the job of transporting fats into our mitochondria for burning.

A meta-analysis of randomized trials suggests that L-carnitine improves patient outcomes.
Specifically, it exerts an effect on hypertension, oxidative stress, nitric oxide, and inflammation.

A further systematic review found that L-carnitine is associated with a 27% reduction in all-cause mortality in heart failure patients.

A systematic review shows that higher L-carnitine intake in type 2 diabetes patients improves fasting glucose levels and the overall cholesterol profile. And According to a systematic review and meta-analysis of nine randomized controlled trials, subjects using L-carnitine supplementation lost

"significantly more weight" than the control group

Glutathione

Commonly known as the 'master antioxidant,' glutathione has a score of research linking it to
Anti-aging benefits
Increasing longevity
Preventing illness
Reducing the risk of chronic disease
Strengthening the immune system
It helps protect every cell in our body from cellular damage, which can lead to many chronic diseases.
As a result, keeping glutathione levels high is important for our overall health
Endogenous Glutathione Production

First of all, our body produces glutathione endogenously. In other words, our body uses raw materials (in this case: amino acids) to make glutathione.

For this process to occur, we should have adequate levels of the amino acids cysteine, glutamate, and glycine.
These amino acids are known as glutathione precursors, and each of these amino acids is present in beef. On the positive side, beef also contains a reasonably high source of complete (pre-formed) dietary glutathione.

Beef is high in minerals:
Calcium, Copper, Iron, magnesium, manganese, Potassium, Phosphorus, Selenium and zinc.

And while all these are important to base life and body function – iron deficiency anemia deserves a mention of its own.

Sadly, iron deficiency anemia is a growing epidemic around the world.
In a developed country such as the United States, nutrient deficiencies shouldn't be a cause of death, yet anemia kills thousands every year.
To be exact, the latest release of statistics showed that Anemia hospitalized 146,000 Americans in one year. 5,219 of these people died

Globally it's even worse, and according to the World Health Organization, 1.62 billion people suffer from iron deficiency anemia

A word on Heme and Non-Heme Iron
There are two types of iron available in food, and we refer to them as heme and non-heme iron.
Heme Iron: Heme iron is the most bioavailable form of iron, and meat and other animal foods exclusively contain it.

Non-Heme Iron: Non-heme iron is found in plant foods such as fruit, vegetables, and nuts.
In comparison to heme iron, our body finds it more difficult to absorb.

One of the best health benefits of beef meat is that it contains a substantial amount of heme iron. That combined with the fact that beef has a full load of B vitamins makes for good uptake of iron and helps with energy, sleeping and repair of the body.

Carnosine

Carnosine reduces the harms of a process called 'glycation' which involves advanced glycation end-products (AGES).

Glycation is central to the aging process and progressively damages our body, potentially leading to atherosclerosis and various other chronic diseases

Additionally, carnosine helps boost the immune system and reduce inflammation. The amino acid is also thought to help prevent lipid peroxidation within our cells.

All making it a solid choice and an original human food.

Notes on cooking proteins:

Never use tenderizers or cook anything in bags or use tinfoil. You can cook in the over, crock pot or stove top in a ceramic fry pan – no teflon!
Use only olive oil or butter when frying.

Do not deep fry, avoid breading proteins.

Note: Other meats that can be cooked at a temperature are also ok to eat like: lamb, venison and other game meat.

Remember - Pork, chicken, shellfish and shrimp are not human food. You can not eat them raw or at temperature.
Sorry, I know bacon is yummy but it's off the menu.

How much should we eat?

This brings us to -

2nd Rule of shopping
Count the heads

The truth is if you compare the number of heads of all the livestock to the number of heads of lettuces, broccoli and other vegetables - you would see that the vegetables win, at least 4 to 1.

So when we eat it should be 4 vegetable to one protein. The green should be the biggest part of the meal, even breakfast. I know, I know, green at breakfast? Yes!
I get to the whole breakfast mess in a few pages, for now just remember- lots of greens.

As always with greens comes the question, raw or cooked? Well as much raw as possible then steamed for the rest.
As a rule start with 30% raw- 70% steamed. Then work to reverse those percentages.

Eating over cooked greens, juicing greens and ice burg lettuces is does not count.

We need the whole green vegetable, as close to its original form as possible.

Somewhere along the way we got lost, we started mixing up fruits with vegetables! I'm not too sure how it happened but it did.

They are not interchangeable, fruit does not have any of the fibers, plant fats or nutrients that most vegetables have in them.

Yes I know that the fruit is yummy but you need your vegetables at every meal.

3Rd rule of shopping
Dairy is a garnish!

No one would have to avoid dairy products
if they would use them in very small
doses. Cheese is not a meal; it is not a
third of a meal. Cheese should be used as
some use salt, just a shake.
You will not need cream in your coffee,
because you will not be drinking anything
but water.
Do not drink milk! Or do but know that it
has no real value anymore.
Please do not feed it to your children; they
need pure water just like you. However, if
you choose to use milk buy only organic
milk and buy the whole milk, at least you
might get some medium change fats that
can be of benefit and the fat will stabilize
your blood sugar.

NOTE; although located in the dairy
section of the store - eggs are not dairy!
please eat only organic eggs.
Also eat the whole egg, not just the
whites.
No, it will not raise blood lipids.
Do not eat Eggbeater, they are loaded
with carbohydrates and are not found in
nature.

Now a word about yogurt - Yogurt can be of benefit, if you eat only plain, nature, organic yogurt.

Also, Greek yogurt is great - high in protein and lower in carbohydrates. You can add fresh berries and nuts.
Anything else is a waste of time and money.
 Do not be fooled by yogurt coated nuts, frozen yogurt treats or TCBY, this stuff is not good for anyone.
It is not better for you either.

I get that argument all the time.
"It's better than eating ice cream".

It's like saying speed is better for you than cocaine.
It is a dumb point of view we use to rationalize bad food choices.
Do not kid yourself; they're both loaded with sugar of one form or another.

Both have been processed to ensure no nutritional value and using either will only continue the cravings for sweets that plague our diets.

4th rule of shopping
Buy nuts and seeds

Do not make a meal out of either, but include them in your diet. They are rich in healthy fats, protein and low glycemic carbohydrates.

Do not eat roasted nuts of any kind, they are bad fat now! Roasting nuts turns the good oil in nuts into free radicals and then most of the benefit is gone. Also, no salt! Stop it, try to eat stuff for the taste of the product – not the stuff we can put on it.

Please do not be afraid of the fat in nuts. These fats are great to stabilize your blood sugar and are heart healthy.
Also, the fat in nuts helps to reduce cravings. If you are craving sweets (you did not eat enough at your last meal but anyway) take a tablespoon of nut butter or a few whole (un roasted nuts) and wait a few minutes.

The intake of the fat will release a hormone called CCK that tells the brain that we are satisfied and to stop craving.

Also nut butters are ok, but in small doses. Buy only organic nut butters, ground fresh is best. Keep nut butters refrigerated, the oil in nuts can turn from a positive to a negative if exposed to heat. Free radicals can develop even at room temps.
Do not use nuts or nut butters in cooking or baking for the same reason.

Lastly do not replace any real protein for nut – they have way more fat than protein.
Most importantly – Peanuts are NOT NUTS – they are beans

 And PLEASE stay away from these new fat free peanut butter powders – how could that be good for you –
It is - say it with me...   NOT FOUND IN NATURE!

5th rule of shopping
Cooking oils

As a rule, you want to use the oven for cooking, the burner for steaming and the frying pan for quick stir-fry only. Use nothing but olive oil or grape seed oil for the latter.

I am about to kill a holy cow of the health food industry- canola oil. Not because of some mainstream anti-health reports or because I do not understand that the harmful effects of rapeseed have been removed.

I kill the Canola oil cow because it could not be found in nature before the seed chemists made it.
Hybrid plants and vegetables are not found naturally.
Also, Canola oil has very low resistances to free radical production - making it a bad choice.
Do not use any products made with Canola oil.
Not salad dressings or baked goods or ANYTHING WITH CANOLA OIL IN IT.

Soy and vegetable oils are also bad for cooking.
And never buy any oil in a spray can even from a health food store (they do have pumps that work on air pressure alone which are great) but no aerosols.

If olive oil or grape seed oil is not available, use butter.

Never use any butter look-a- likes, I can't believe it's not butter should be named "It's worse than butter".

In the end use only a small amount of cooking oil, never use it as garnish and use half as much as vinegar in salad dressing.

Note; there is a new produce made with yogurt to try and fool you, don't be fooled. It is just as bad as the rest.

6th rule of shopping
Rotate fruits

If you recall we talked about counting the heads of livestock and the heads of vegetables.
With fruit it is a little tricky.
First, fruit plants and trees are out matched by the vegetables 8 to 1.

Second, fruit seasons are shorter than most vegetables.

Third, fruit has a very short window of ripeness when it can be consumed.

And last but not least, while fructose does not induce the same insulin response as other sugars, it does keep that sweet taste craving going.

Common sense tells us then that fruit should be used in moderation.

Two to four pieces a day and trying to choose the low glycemic fruits (see list) .

Juice is not the same thing as fruit.

When we juice, we process - juice is not found in nature.
Sorry juice guy! We do need the pulp and the pectin fiber from fruit. Also fruit in smoothies or shake is not the same as fruit.

Please do not let anyone tell you that they have a pill that is like getting 5 servings of fruit.
I got trapped for a whole day with one of these juice pill people at an expo, it was horrifying.
The whole pitch on these pills is that you can use them, if you cannot eat all the fruit you need.
This is as bad as the Atkins diet that keeps you away from vegetables, both are crazy - And a lie.
You need to eat food, real food.

7th Rule of shopping
Read labels

As I pointed out in our field trip to the store, things are not what they seem. When picking meats, you must look at the label. If it has a list of solutions that are injected into the meat...do not buy it. These solutions are to make the meat tender, last longer and to make the meat look more appealing.

Any and all meat should not have an ingredient label on it, if it does – think twice about buying it!!!

Most for these solutions are sodium based. All are man made. Also if you see the Radua (the same symbol used to mark radioactive material) this indicates that the food has been treated with low level radiation. Do I need to tell you....run - do not walk.

We live in a to-go world
So much so that groceries have taken to seasoning fresh meats, chicken etc..

So all you have to do is throw it in the pan or oven.
Do not buy these things.

They look great and seem like a time saver but in the end – you're much better off preparing your own food with fresh – natural seasoning and herbs.

And – the prepared fully cooked stuff they are making looks good too but, avoid it. They will not be taking the time to use the best ingredients, natural oils and your paying top dollar for a cooked meal that has been refrigerated – if I invited you over and fed you food I made two days ago – we'd call that Leftovers!

In the produce department, if you do not want to buy only organic vegetables, buy only fruits and vegetables that are farmed in the U.S.A.

This will only ensure that you get FDA approved pesticides, not much comfort.

You will need to look at the list on the most treated and sprayed crops (see list section) to avoid these or use a vegetable wash that can be found at any health food store.

As above – the stores now are pre-cutting vegetables for you to make your life easier (and shorter).

All vegetables should be cut fresh when your cooking!!!
Plus even using a natural stabilizer like lemon juice (used to keep cut apples from turning brown) is breaking down the food and reducing the benefits.

A word on frozen foods

Do not buy them.

No, I mean this, do not buy them.
The bio availability of the vitamins is reducing by freezing.
Also, with vegetable, the minerals will not be absorbed by your body.
Same with fruits - do not waste your money. And do your best to not get sucked into the falsehood of

"its better than nothing"

its not and - we do not make these trade-offs!

Always remember the envelopes, we want the 100's!
As for all other types of frozen foods, dinners and meats, they have all the solution you need to kill you and none of the nutrition.

A word on the deli

None of the meat you find in the deli can be found in that form in nature.
It is true that you can find some small, independently owned delis and stores that still roast a round of beef or cook a ham and then slice it for you but these places are few and far between.

Today, most places are using the same chipped, formed and pressed meat. All of it is over processed and injected and flavored to make it taste like the thing you could get from just using the real product in its real form.

 Why do they do it? MONEY!

And to make it easy for you... In all these "ease products" we miss something very important.
Something we understand in every other facet of our lives.

I call it -
THE QUALITY OF TIME
The idea that things of quality take time is not new and in most cases it seems stupid to even point it out – we know this to be true.
Yet with food?
We simple do not think that way.

Fast food is the best example of this. By its name alone, they are telling you that it is not a quality product – we just are not listening.

 No one would be comfortable on the plane if we knew they did the inspection in 2 minute! Or used cheaper parts to stay on schedule.

As for the cheese, read the label, buy in small amounts, use as a garnish only.
By the way; they love it in the deli, when you ask them to let you see the label.
With a look of confusion, the counter person will pull out the product and put it on the counter for you to look at.

Buy only naturally aged cheese with no coloring. As a rule, just avoid the regular grocery store deli.

If you do not want to buy from the health food store, buy the Cabot cheese brand. It is all natural and available at almost any store.

8th rule of shopping
No desert

The main taste we have developed in this
country is the sweet taste.
This has to stop.
Ending the meal by eating something
sweet just adds to the blood sugar spike.

This will cause digestive problems and you
will undo a lot of the good you did with
your good food choices (this is true even
with fruit).

If you must have a sweet thing – eat it
between meals and make it something
small and satisfying like chocolate.

Never buy sugar free products or fake
sugar.
Never use low fat sweets – the fat in
sweets help to reduce the blood sugar
spike – so milk chocolate is better for you
then dark.
I know this is in direct opposition to the
conventional wisdom of the day but your
not really getting any benefit from that
dark chocolate.

Its not a human food – so you must
choose the lesser of evils here and the
lesser evils are lower glycemic product's
like: milk chocolate, full fat ice cream and
some fruit.

Never buy anything with corn syrup or bad
oils.
Never get low calorie sweets.
Stay away from cakes, donuts, baked
goods and pies.

We need to understand how important the
food we choose to put in us is and why we
have to do it.

CHAPTER THREE

Putting it all together -
cause, you got to eat!

RATIO OF FOOD FOR EACH MEAL

As a rule, use this simple ratio chart to eat.

 One full plate of raw salad and the other with 25% of the plate filled with healthy (human) proteins and the rest of the plate steamed vegetables – 3 times a day.

Its not very scientific but its a good guideline. Yes every meal....even breakfast.
The truth is that we are still eating our morning meal like its the 1800s!

Back then we did not have a way to stabilize food. We ate grains (now known as bread or cereal) and we ate fresh eggs (from under the chicken) or salted meat (bacon or ham).
This was a full meal of necessity!!!

Today we have a full range of food open to us and these habits are just that – habits!

There is no proof that humans need less nutrients in the morning.

In fact, the reverse is true, there is no other time during the 24 hour day that we need more nutrient than in the morning.

We eat our last meal around 6-8pm the day before then go to bed. We sleep 8 hours.
During the night we rebuild cells, make human growth hormone and replenish the body.
We wake in the morning (having gone a minimum of 12 hours without food) in need of a lot of stuff and our answer to this is ????

A muffin and a cup of coffee! Or tons of carb and sugar or worse…...NOTHING!

Breakfast is important.

You must have a good meal to recover from the 12 hour (or longer) fast!

In fact, it is called BREAK FAST! For this reason.

MAKE DAILY DEPOSITS

One of the best ways to keep a business going is to have a steady stream of cash going into the bank every day or even better a few times a day.
Why? Because you have bills to pay.
Think of your body as a business. And in a very real sense – think of your body as a manufacturing business – because it is.

Everything in a manufacturing operation depends on four things
1) raw material on hand
2) energy and motivation of the labor force
3) all systems running optimally
4) a clean, safe and productive work place

Every minute of every day you replace thousands of cells, you remove old bone and rebuild it, you produce energy and hormones that run every system in your body and you clean and detoxify.

Why would we ever believe that we do not need the raw material to complete these jobs?
Its all in the way you look at things.

You have to start thinking of the body in this way. Your body does most of these things without you ever knowing its happening.
Yet we will stave it, deprive it of a food cash flow.

This type of behavior leads to a reduction of the quality of our lives in three ways;

1) Lack of energy. The sluggish feeling in the morning and the mid afternoon nappy time that almost everyone feels and have come to accept is the by-product of not getting what your body needs.

2) Lack of sleep. We can't get to sleep or can't stay asleep is all related to food.
3) Reduce longevity. When we do not have enough material coming in the body – we can not rebuild and replenish the body cells,

Further, nutrient deficiencies, slowed brain function and reduced productivity are all accelerated by the body not being able to function optimally.
Skipping meals, having low nutrient meals and/or loading with sugar for quick energy all cause multiple issues.

Ranging from hormone and blood sugar imbalances to aches and pains and are the road to disease.

Think of the clock – so we eat a good balanced dinner at 7pm.
Then we sleep and get up at 7am.

Then we go until noon without anything of value.
That's 17 hours without a bite of anything that we really need.
Then we have a high starch meal with little in the way of nutrient.
This causes our body to go from empty to a full on blood sugar tidal wave. Then we feel tried and sleepy in the afternoon and by dinner we have exhausted the body.

We have reduced our metabolic rate and then we slam the body full again and then do nothing for four hours and then sleep some more.

We are not making the deposits on time and the bank bags are only half full.
Its just bad business.

So we need those 3 deposits a day – evenly spaced and full of nutrient.

Often people will say to me that it seems like too much work to always be on point with food. That if they can not eat what they want – whats the point in life?

The one I love the most is that they simply can not live without this type of food or thing or junk food. I have taken to explaining it this way.
Its not that you can't live without it – its that you will not choose to. And while I can admire the stance on the yummy things you love, the truth is that its not like your giving up an arm or a child…..its just a Coke or a twinkie!

In many ways the argument for eating crap is like a drug addict.

We exchange 3 – 30 minute eating sessions of bliss for 22 hours of torture. While speaking about it like its a quality of life issue.
Eating is not our life – its the thing that provides us with life.

 We should be enjoying the rest of the day.
No one ever drove across the country and only took pictures of the gas stations they stopped at to fill up (imagine that slide show?).

Or raved about the time spent on line buying the tickets to Hawaii and said nothing about the trip!
Its just insane that we think that way but most of us do.

Not to beat the horse but I have even compared it to going to a strip club.

You waste money on girls that you will never have any relationship with (and if you could...would you want too?).

Instead of directing your time and energy into building real, healthy relationships. Sure, it could be something you do once or twice a year but ask anyone – if you go to that club everyday – they will tell you that you have a real problem.

CHAPTER 4

A LITTLE MORE DETAIL

So, we have the basics.
Eat 3 times a day, sleep and fill the body with nutrient – not crap.
Enjoy the 22.5 hours of the day and do not trade off your health for a quick yummy fix.
But there has to more?

Yes, there is. As we move forward we must also look at the activity levels, body size and any health issues that need to be addressed.

Activity is the first, and the most misunderstood part.
There are simple and age old saying that are just so true its silly. My favorite one is that

A body in motion stays in motion.

So stays in motion, we need to move.
Every movement we do puts a load on the body.

These movements are interpreted by the body as signals that we need to build and maintain muscle and bone density.
They help us burn fat and calories and keep us fit.
With that said – its very important to eat for your activity levels and customize the meals and intake to make sure that we are not in a deficit or over drawing the bank account.
The best way to get a baseline of what you need in terms of the macro nutrients (protein, green carbs and fat) is to get your body fat percentage.
We are trying to do 2 things at once.

1) Feed the body so that we do not lose lean body mass during exerciser.
You can lose weight on the scale but still be fat.
I know this seems counter intuitive but its true.
Your metabolic rate (the amount of calories you burn at rest) is one of the most important things to care for.
We keep this high by keeping lean body mass and muscles mass.

Too many fad or concept diets are only interested in taking what I call "scale weight" off your body.

These diets do not care about the lean body mass.
 Most are only designed to remove water weight and then start burning as much weight as possible no matter if its muscle or fat. These diets are by nature – unhealthy.

They will get you down a few sizes but after – you will have less muscle, a lower metabolic rate and you will put weight back on even faster then you did before.
 This yo-yo dieting is the foundation of every mass marketed diet out there. You know someone right now that will say.

"I went on this diet and lost 20 pounds but I gained it all back"

That was not a successful business.

Its like looking at your balance in the account and saying "I've got 10K in there – I'm rich!" but by the end of the week when the bills are paid – they are broke.

Any real and solid weight loss plan will make you check your body fat and lean body mass and plan a diet to insure that you only lose fat.
Which after all is what we really want to do.

So we check the body mass all the time and adjust the intake to keep the body working optimally and moving in the right direction of fat burning.

2) Keep energy levels and metabolic rate high in order to burn off fat. When we do not keep the right amounts of macro nutrients coming in the body during movement the body runs out of fuel. But it can not just stop so it strips lean mass from muscles and organs for energy.

Lowering the lean mass and over time this type of bad burn can lead to quite a few health problems.

Think of it this way.
You need a good fire in the fireplace to keep your family warm.
So you need wood or a full tank of oil to keep that fire lit. The food is the wood or oil. If you do not keep that flowing – you end up pulling wood from the walls to stoke the fire until you have holes in the house.
It is the law of diminishing return.
Over my 20 years in natural health as an educator and consultant, I have performed over 40 thousand tests on people from all walks of life.

What I know from these tests is that you can be 120 lbs and have 35% body fat and you can be 220 lbs and have 15% body fat.

The point is that looking thin is not, in any way, a good judge of a persons health.

Most of these people that are known as "skinny fat".

They are right where the chart says they should be for their height and body frame but they have little energy, lower immune function and given the right set of circumstances can pound on weight quickly.
Whereas the 220 pound person with 15% body fat may present as someone that is over the range as far as some chart says.

However, they have plenty of energy, muscle mass and a high metabolic rate that is all keeping them healthier then most people.
And lets not forget that weight not withstanding, What we really are looking for here is health.

We need to also remember that whatever we are doing – we have to find a way to keep it going.

If you starve and lose "scale weight" you will never be free from the yo-yo effect.

You will always be going up and down and live your life on some type of "diet cycle". Most of us, myself included, have longed for that mystical body that we see others have and have openly said,

"I wish I did not have to always worry about gaining weight"

Well its not a mystical gift that these people have been given from the gods. It is something that you can build. It is a combination of habits, metabolic rate and proper food intake – its science, not alchemy.

The first step is keeping the body's metabolic rate high and the muscle mass in place.

It is a balancing act but it is not too hard once we understand how things work.

So lets have some examples;

a 200 pound person has 30% (or 60 pounds of fat) so their lean body mass is 140 pounds.

If they have a basic metabolic rate and do nothing other than their regular activity – they will need:
70 grams of protein a day
30 grams of healthy fats a day
Unlimited green carbs a day
To keep their body running right and not lose muscle mass.
That is a half gram of protein per one pound of lean body mass and a quarter gram of healthy fat per pound of lean body mass.

½ gram protein per 1 lbs of LBM (lean body mass)

¼ gram healthy fats per 1 lbs of LBM.

Green carbohydrates are not counted.
If this person works out 45 minutes per day – 3 times per week the numbers are increased by 25%.

If they do this 5 times a week – the number are increased 30%.

By monitoring the lean body mass & eating the human foods – we can navigate the mess that is weight loss with relative ease. And avoid "wasting" (losing muscle mass for a quick down tick on the scale.

**BODY SIZE
The ultimate flash over substance
issue!**

Lets talk about skeletal frame….you've got one and its really all yours.

No two are alike and even in twins – the frame size and weight can vary.

Comparing your body to others is a huge waste of time and can be dangerous. Many a young person have been driven to near death and damaged their health trying to look like someone else.
We need to be realistic in what we want or rather what we can have.
 The average skeletal weight is around 12 – 15% of your total weight (or rather your idea weight).
So, if you are in the "healthy weight" for your height then a 150.00 pound person will have 18 - 22.5 pounds of bones.
Sounds simple enough right?….

Nope!

What we have found is that heavy people – those at 33% body fat never get osteoporosis.

Why?... because the body is a response system.
The more weight your body has on it or the more you lift – the bigger and stronger the bones get.
Hence the term – big boned!
If you have been overweight during your bone development time (0 – 29 years of age) -you might have bigger bones than others, albeit by only a point or two.
It might not matter much in the general scheme of things but it might stop you from getting "skinny jeans" on or that tight cut jacket.

Does this mean your fat? No.

However..you could lose all the weight you want and still look like your packed in your suit.

Also, for every pound of weight you gain and carry for a time – your body will build muscle to carry the load.
 And so, your muscle mass will increase even if your over weight. Many people have an "abstract body goal" that closely resembles what you looked like in high school or college.
Your body has changed since then and trying to get there would be impossible.

Lastly, muscle weights more than fat....so even trying to get back to your "then" weight – might be impossible or at least – ill advised.
Since you'd have to lose muscle to get there.

The point is – making reasonable goals for your NOW body makes the most sense. And always remember – health is the goal....
   I'm only talking about this because most of the time if you move to the human diet – you will lose fat as a natural by-product of eating right.
You just have to be careful not to get sucked into the "I'm going to be skinny" rabbit hole.

WATER

Its so important that I should have started with
it on page one – water is a huge part of the human diet. Water and how much we should drink of it is by far one of the least understood and overlooked aspects of our health.

We have been told everything from:
"It doesn't matter"
to
"8 – 8 oz. Glasses a day" neither is true.

Your body is not water tight. You leak all the time and you use water in the production of many products inside.

Which is to say that even if you are not working out or sweating – you are using up water.

Water is needed for everything. From absorption of vitamins and minerals to the production of enzymes that help you digest and produce hormones.
The texture of our skin and the cleaning of the body.

Brain function, liver function and elimination all depend on water. If we were to look at it from an order of priorities for life itself – the list would look like this:

Air
Water
Food

As a rule, we need about 3 oz. of pure water every half hour of waking hours each day. If you're up 16 hours – you should be able to take in about 96 oz a day with little to no problems.
 Slow and steady intake drops the times to the bathroom and ensures that you get enough in without any risk of over hydration.

The water should be pure and in a perfect world – distilled.

Do not listen to people that say that distilled water is dead! The whole planet runs on distillation!
Water is heated and turned into vapor.

That vapor is pure and free from heavy metals and minerals as it rises and then is returned to the ground in the form of rain.

This is how everything grows –
everywhere!
Crops of trees get their minerals from the
ground and water from the sky.

So, drink distilled water for hydration and
eat vegetables and natural "human" foods
for your minerals.
You also get minerals from the air!

I know it sounds crazy but it's true. Living
close to the ocean – you breath in ionized
minerals from the air.

I love when someone tells me that they do
not like the taste of water.
Water should have no taste!

If your water has a "taste" it's because its
got something in it that does not belong
there!
Tap water has a taste!
It tastes like crap.
Because its not pure water – its "treated"
water.
A combination of bad ideas, chemicals and
bacteria killers that is piped into your
home as if that is how things should be.

My two favorite poisons added to water
are Fluoride and Chlorine.

Fluoride

"The effects of fluoride on various aspects of endocrine function should be examined, particularly with respect to a possible role in the development of several diseases or mental states in the United States. Major areas of investigation include; thyroid disease (especially in light of decreasing iodine intake by the U.S. population)," the National Research Council concluded in 2006.

Countries around the world have walked back their support of Fluoride in the water supply and in toothpaste.
Fluoride is a neurotoxin that passes through the "brain blood barrier" into our brains and it passes through the placenta and can effect the fetus's brain development. And most of the added Fluoride is not natural.
Check this one out:
Sodium Fluoride (NaF), a constituent of most toothpastes, has been used as the active ingredient in insecticides, wood preservatives, fungicides and rat poison.

It works on rats by causing lesions in their stomachs which eventually result in the rat bleeding to death - just the thing to put in our mouths, then!

If you have children, you probably find it difficult to stop them from ingesting some of their toothpaste, especially as it has been made to be tasty to encourage brushing. But what could it be doing to their bodies?

On every tube this warning is there: WARNING: KEEP OUT OF REACH OF CHILDREN UNDER SIX YEARS OF AGE. IN CASE OF ACCIDENTAL OVERDOSE, SEEK PROFESSIONAL ASSISTANCE OR CONTACT A POISON CONTROL CENTER IMMEDIATELY

In 1992 a randomized double-blind study was conducted in which healthy male volunteers were given either sodium fluoride or sodium monofluorophosphate (MFP) tablets (both common ingredients in toothpaste) for seven days.

Before the trial, both sets of volunteers had their stomach linings assessed. This was repeated again at the end of the trial.

"Those in the MFP group showed no significant changes but seven out of ten in the Sodium Fluoride group had significant stomach lesions, including acute haemorrhages and free blood in their stomachs".

(Gastroenterology 1992; 30: 252-4)

And, World renowned toxicologist, Dr Samuel Epstein states that "the use of fluoride in toothpaste is controversial because of suggestive evidence of carcinogenicity"

Other issues with the use of Fluoride are:

Kidney Toxicity
Renal excretion is the main elimination route for inorganic fluoride from your body.
As a consequence, the cells of your kidney are exposed to relatively high concentrations of fluoride, making your kidneys vulnerable to fluoride toxicity.

According to the Subcommittee on Health Effects of Ingested Fluoride of the National Research Council, animal studies have demonstrated that exposure to fluoride at concentrations of 100 to 380 milligrams per liter of drinking water can cause swelling in between the kidney tubules, dilation of renal tubules and death of proximal and renal tubules. I.Q. deficits
A meta-analysis of 27 studies linked fluoride ingestion to I.Q. deficits in children, notes the Fluoride Action Network.

Three studies from China have discovered that the increased intake of fluoride during pregnancy can harm the fetal brain.

Animal and human research show that ingesting excess fluoride aggravates the effects of iodine deficiency.
 Iodine is essential for proper thyroid function. Inadequate intake of iodine during infancy and early childhood can lead to permanent brain damage, including mental retardation.

And for those that still argue that its needed for healthy teeth:
Dental Flurossis
Consuming too much fluoride in early childhood when teeth are developing under the gums can lead to dental fluorosis.
This condition is characterized by failure of tooth enamel to crystallize properly leading to defects such as brittleness, staining that is barely noticeable to severe brown stains and surface pitting.
The severity of dental fluorosis depends on factors such as the dose, timing and duration of fluoride consumption. Children aged 0 to 8 years are at risk for developing dental fluorosis, because this is when permanent teeth begin to form under the gums.

Chlorine

In the 1970's it was discovered that chlorine, when added to water, forms Trihalomethanes (chlorinated by-products) by combining with certain naturally occurring organic matter such as vegetation and algae.

In 1992 the American Journal of Public Health published a report that showed a 15% to 35% increase in certain types of cancer for people who consume chlorinated water.

This report also stated that much of these effects were due to showering in chlorinated water. (more on that in personal environment ahead)
The National Cancer Institute estimates cancer risks for people who consume chlorinated water to be 93% higher than for people who do not. The effects of drinking chlorinated water have been debated for decades.

However, most experts now agree that there are some significant risks related to consuming chlorine and chlorinated by-products.

CHLORINATED WATER CAN AFFECT CANCER RISK
Epidemiology 1998;9(1):21-28,29-35

Lifetime consumption of chlorinated tap water can more than double the risk of bladder and rectal cancers in certain individuals, two new studies conclude.

Both studies examined the lifetime water-consumption patterns, diets and lifestyles of over 2,200 middle-aged and elderly Iowans suffering from either bladder, colon, or rectal cancers. Those profiles were then compared with those of a pool of nearly 2,000 healthy 'controls'.

The link between chlorine and bladder and rectal cancers has long been known. Only recently have researchers found a link between common chlorine disinfectant and breast cancer.

 Breast cancer affects one out of every eight American women. A recent study conducted in Hartford, Connecticut found that women with breast cancer have 50-60 percent higher levels of organochlorines (chlorine by-products) in their breast tissue than cancer-free women.

So, the point is - we should not be drinking this stuff.

It should not be in our water or used in our mouths and advocates of insanity will tell you that it is fine to drink.

However, the very fact there is so much junk in the water that there is a multi billion dollar industry that does nothing but remove that crap should prove my point. If there was nothing but water in your water – they would be out of business.

You have been lied to about this forever. Told that all water is the same and only "fools" and "Health Nuts" fall for this pure water nonsense!

Anyone that attempts to sell you this argument should be dismissed from their job and possible prosecuted.

Your mechanic will not tell you to use "any oil" or "any gas" or 'any tires" for your car! Why?
Because your car (a far simpler design than your body) is designed with very specific needs to run optimally.

Try submitting plans for a home that use
"any type" of building materials.

Make the argument to the planning
department that all building materials are
the same.
Tell these professionals that they are crazy
to believe that one thing is better then
another – you'll be asked to leave that
office.

**There is only a few truths out there
and
"Source and purity matter" is one of
them.**

R/O water is a close seconds to distillation
and can be found everywhere today.

This is also true when someone tells you
that you get "water" or "hydration" from
drinking anything. Like coffee, tea and
beer are all made from water! If you run
into one of these crazies – be polite but
get away fast!

But if do not care about any of that and
still think water is a choice rather than a
necessity, I'll give you a best reason to
drink pure water.

Weight gain!

Often people think that they are hungry but they are really just in need of a drink of water.
This can often lead to over eating and also over time change the way we automatically respond to the thirst signals.

Drinking coffee or tea or alcohol will remove water from our systems and create the need for more hydration.

Digestion and elimination all depend on us staying well hydrated.

Absent of proper hydration we do not absorb vitamins and minerals or properly burn fat. This, in turn, cause us to gain weight and feel bad. Starting a downward spiral that leads to low muscle mass, low energy, fat retention and a slow and painful end filled with suffering.

That should get you thinking & drinking!

Personal Environment

We simply can not overlook this last
detail. Mainly because it is one of last big
lies that keep us from being healthy.

What we breath in and use on our bodies
is just as important as the food and water
we put inside it.

I want to start here with one great fact....

Before the mid 1940's – we had a little
less than 5000 patents for chemicals and
then by the mid 1950's we had over
50,000!

And since then we have added thousands
more. These things had permanent our
world and our lives. They are in everything
from the ground we grow in, the water we
drink to the air we breath.
Yet there are still people and agencies that
will tell you that it had no effect on us or
our world.

It's a little like me coming over to your home and pulling down walls, removing doors and blocking up you access to your bathroom and then calling you a fool for thinking that it will have any effect on your life!

A lot of books and reports have be very clear about the fact that your home can be 100 times more toxic then the outside air but no one is listening.

In the chapter before we covered that the body is not water tight and that we can breath in way more toxins from the hot water then you can get from drinking.

So, why would no one tell you to stop adding more crap to your inside air?

And why would anyone tell you that it doesn't matter?
We have been so confused and lied to so much that we have no sense of priorities in this area.

Case in point are people that in an outdoor air environment like a park will complain about someone smoking but we will use bleach on everything in our home, plug in chemical air fresheners that out gas every second of the day.

Spray all of our things with Febreze while using chemical dryer sheets that have so much chemicals in them that you can smell them outside your home from the dryer vent.

On top of that we get in the shower with that poison hot water and cover our bodies from head to toe with chemicals that range from alcohol and petrolatum to known carcinogens like polypropylene glycol.
Later we cover our armpits with aluminum and cover our faces with more petrolatum and chemicals.

We all know that the dermis (our skin) – is the biggest organ in the body and that we absorb right through it but we do nothing about it.

We think nothing about it and we have been told to not worry about it. Well we have not been told this here in the US – however....its not the same in other countries in the world.

 In fact there are 1100 chemicals that are used in body care products in the US that are banned in the EU since 2011!

you can look them up at:
https://eur-lex.europa.eu/LexUriServ/
LexUriServ.do?
uri=CONSLEG:1976L0768:20100301:en:P
DF

The report is 163 pages long and the list
of banned products starts on page 18 and
is 47 pages long!!!!!! I have a condensed
list next.

Meanwhile on this side of the Atlantic -
our FDA has banned 9 of these
products!!!!!

What we are told by our government is
that every other 1st world country in the
world is crazy and we just know better!

This type of American - centric argument
is replete in all forms of research in our
country. From drugs to pesticide to food
additives to chemicals.

No one else anywhere in the world can do
research and that if it is not done here – it
simply is not worth believing.

It would be funny if it was not so
dangerous.

And it does not stop once you leave the house, your lawn is sprayed with toxic chemicals, your car is plastics that out gas in the heat and on top of that we spray the car or hang chemical air freshers in the form of a pine tree from the rear view!!!!
More recently they have clip-on air freshers that you attach to the A/C vents so just in case your not getting enough toxicity from the ambient air – they can be blown right in your face!!!

You have control of all of these thing! And you should exercise that control. I can think of nothing more counterproductive than buying all organic food and pure drinking water, working out and taking care of your body while poisoning yourself in other ways. Its a waste of time, money and life. Its not just self destructive, it's insane!

SO CLEAN HOUSE! TODAY.

Get rid of these things and save money and your health.
You can keep a clean house and a fresh smelling house without the use of chemicals.

By using clean and green products that are readily available just about everywhere these days.

See the next pages for the list of big bad guys.

Chemicals in your personal environment that must go!

1,4-dioxane

Nearly half of the cosmetics containing ethoxylated surfactants have been shown to contain 1,4-dioxane.
FROM THE MSDS
1,4-dioxane may exert its effects through inhalation, skin absorption, and ingestion. 1,4-dioxane is listed as a carcinogen, causes cancer.
EFFECTS OF OVEREXPOSURE:
1,4-dioxane is an eye and mucous membrane irritant, primary skin irritant, central nervous system depressant, nephrotoxin and hepatotoxin. Acute exposure causes irritation, headache, dizziness and narcosis. Chronic inhalation exposure can produce damage to the liver and kidneys and blood disorders. MEDICAL CONDITIONS AGGRAVATED BY EXPOSURE: Preclude from exposure those individuals with diseases of the blood, liver, kidneys, central nervous system and those susceptible to dermatitis.
Also see Ethoxylated surfactants

2-bromo-2-nitropropane-1,3-diol (Bronopol)

Causes allergic contact dermatitis.
Also see
Nitrosating agents

Alcohol, Isopropyl (SD-40)

A solvent that strips away the skin's natural acid layer which protects us from bacteria, moulds and viruses. It is made from propylene, a petroleum bi-product and is thought to promote brown spots and premature aging of skin.

Anionic Surfactants

Anionic refers to the negative charge these surfactants have. They may be contaminated with nitrosamines, which are carcinogenic. Surfactants can pose serious health threats.
They are used in car washes, as garage floor cleaners and engine degreasers - and in the majority of personal care products that foam.
Anionic Surfactants include the following:
Ammonium Laureth Sulfate (ALES)
Ammonium Lauryl Sulfate (ALS)
Disodium Dioctyl Sulfosuccinate
Disodium Laureth Sulfosuccinate

Disodium Oleamide Sulfosuccinate
Laureth or Lauryl Sulfate
Lauryl or Cocoyl Sarcosine
Potassium Coco Hydrolysed Collagen
Sodium Cocoyl Sarcosinate
Sodium Laureth Sulfate (SLES)
Sodium Lauroyl Sarcosinate
Sodium Lauryl Sulfate (SLS)
Sodium Methyl Cocoyl Taurate
Triethanolamine (TEA)

Benzalkonium Chloride
Primary skin irritant, very toxic chemical.
FROM THE MSDS INGESTION: Material is highly toxic via oral route. If conscious, immediately drink large quantities of fluid to dilute and induce vomiting. Call physician. EFFECTS OF OVEREXPOSURE: Mists can cause irritation to the skin, eyes, nose, throat and mucous membranes. Avoid direct contact.
SYMPTOMS OF OVEREXPOSURE: Muscular paralysis, low blood pressure, central nervous system depression and weakness.
EMERGENCY FIRST AID PROCEDURES: Eyes: Corrosive! Immediately wash eyes with copious amount of water.
INHALATION: Remove person to fresh air. Give oxygen (If breathing is difficult). Call physician.
Also see Cationic Surfactants

Butylated Hudroxyanisole (BHA)

Causes allergic contact dermatitis.

Butylated Hydroxytoluene (BHT)

Causes allergic contact dermatitis.
Contains toluene.
Also see Toluene

Cationic Surfactants
These toxic chemicals have a positive electrical charge. They contain a quaternary ammonium group, often called "quats". Used in hair conditioners, they were originally developed for the paper and fabric industries as softeners and anti-static compounds. With extended usage they can cause hair to become dry and brittle. They are synthetic, irritating, allergenic and toxic chemicals, oral intake can be lethal.

Cationic Sufactants include the following toxic chemicals:
Benzalkonium Chloride
Cetalkonium Chloride
Cetrimonium Chloride
Lauryl Dimonium Hydrolysed Collagen
Stearalkonium Chloride

Chloromethylisothiazolinone

Causes contact dermatitis

Cocoamidopropyl Betaine
FROM THE MSDS

Can cause eye and skin irritation.

DEA (diethanolamine), MEA (Monoethanolamine), and TEA (triethanolamine)

Used in cosmetics to adjust the pH, and used with many fatty acids to convert acid to salt for use as the base for cleansers. TEA causes allergic reactions including eye problems, dryness of hair and skin, and could be toxic if absorbed into the body over a long period of time.
These toxic chemicals are already restricted in Europe due to known carcinogenic effects.
Studies have shown that repeated skin applications of DEA-based detergents resulted in a major increase in the incidence of liver and kidney cancer.
FROM THE MSDS HEALTH HAZARD ACUTE AND CHRONIC: Product is severely irritating to body tissues and possibly corrosive to the eyes.

Amines react with Nitrosating agents to form nitrosamines, which are carcinogenic, causes cancer. Also see Nitrosating agents

Diazolidinyl urea

Contains formaldehyde, a carcinogenic chemical, is a toxic chemical by inhalation, a strong irritant, and causes contact dermatitis.
FROM THE MSDS
SYMPTOMS OF INHALATION:
If misted, will cause irritation of mucous membranes, nose, eyes and throat. Coughing, difficulty breathing.
SYMPTOMS OF SKIN CONTACT: Contact causes smarting and burning sensations, inflammation, burns, and painful blisters. Profound damage to tissue.
SYMPTOMS OF EYE CONTACT:
Will cause painful burning or stinging of eyes and lids, watering of eyes, and inflammation of conjunctiva. Also see Formaldehyde

Dieldrin

A pesticide that has a very long lifespan in water, soil, plants, fish, animals and humans. It has been shown to cause liver cancer in laboratory animals. The US EPA has listed it as a possible human carcinogen. It has been banned in the US since 1974.

However, the International Agency for Research on Cancer has not classified it as a carcinogen.

It is still used in some countries for pest control on cotton and food crops. Prior to 1974 is was also used as a wood preservative to control termites.

There have been studies which have shown reduced liver and immune system function, nervous system effects and indications that it may be an endocrine disruptor.

Human exposure comes mostly from eating meat and fish which have consumed it in water, plants bonemeal food sources.

Dioxins

Dioxins are known to cause cancer and are endocrine disruptors.

There are more than 150 compounds in the dioxin family of compounds and they enter the environment primarily as air pollution.

They are formed as by-products of waste incineration, chemical manufacturing, PVC production, paper bleaching, metal smelting plus a many other industrial processes.

They persist in the environment for decades by attaching to soil particles and sediment in water. They primarily enter the food chain by being in the foods consumed by animals and fish then accumulating in their fatty tissues. Human exposure comes mainly from eating contaminated meat, fish and dairy products.

Formaldehyde
Ethoxylated surfactants
Used in cosmetics as foaming agents, emulsifiers and humectants. As part of the manufacturing process the toxic chemical 1,4-dioxane, a potent carcinogen, is generated.
They are identified in the ingredients by the prefex "PEG", polyethylene, polyethylene glycol, polyoxyethylene, "eth, or oxynol".
Also see
1,4-dioxane
Formaldehyde is a known carcinogen. Causes allergic reactions, irritant and contact dermatitis, headaches and chronic fatigue. The vapor is extremely irritating to the eyes, nose, throat and mucous membranes.
Also see
Nitrosating agents

FD&C color pigments

Synthetic colors made from coal tar. Contain heavy metal salts that deposit toxins onto the skin, causing skin sensitivity and irritation. Animal studies have shown almost all of them to be carcinogenic, can cause cancer.

Fragrance

Fragrance indicates the presence of one of the estimated 4,000 plus separate ingredients, many of which contain phthalates are toxic chemicals and/or carcinogenic.

The FDA reports symptoms which include headaches, dizziness, allergic rashes, skin discoloration, violent coughing and vomiting, and skin irritation. Clinical observation has shown that some fragrances can affect the central nervous system, causing depression, hyperactivity, and irritability.

Imidazolidinyl Urea

The trade name for this toxic chemical is Germall 115. Releases formaldehyde, a carcinogenic chemical, into cosmetics at over 50 degrees Fahrenheit.

Toxic.

Also see

Formaldehyde

Nitrosating agents

Isothiazolinone

Causes contact dermatitis
FROM THE MSDS
EYE CONTACT: Corrosive to the eyes with possible permanent damage.
SKIN CONTACT: Corrosive to the skin, possibly resulting in third degree burns.
 Can be harmful if absorbed, can cause allergic contact dermatitis in susceptible individuals. INGESTION: Can be fatal. INHALATION: Can be corrosive to the mucous membranes and the lungs. Can cause an allergic reaction in susceptible individuals.

Liquidum Paraffinum

Liquidum Paraffinum is just another way to say mineral oil.
Also see
Mineral Oil

Melamine

Melamine has many industrial uses such as when it's combined with other substances such as formaldehyde to make melamin resin.
Melamine was a hot item in the news in early 2007, when veterinary scientists determined it to be the cause of hundreds of dog and cat deaths, because of the unexplained presence of melamine in mass produced dog and cat foods.

Melamine has not nutritional value but it does give a false reading of protein content levels.
Ingestion of melamine can lead to kidney stones and in some cases kidney failure and death.

Methylisothiazolinone and Methylchloroisothiazolinone
Both cause cosmetic allergies

Mineral Oil
Mineral Oil is a petroleum by-product that coats the skin clogging the pores which interferes with skin's ability to eliminate toxins, promoting acne and other disorders.
 Baby oil is 100% mineral oil. Many mineral oil derivatives have been found to be contaminated with cancer causing PAH's (Polycyclic Aromatic Hydrocarbons). Manufacturers use mineral oil because it is extremly inexpensive patroleum byproduct.
Also known as:
Liquidum paraffinum (also known as posh mineral oil!) ,Paraffin oil, Paraffin wax Petrolatum

Nitrosating Agents

There have been concerns expressed world wide about the contamination of cosmetics products with nitrosamines which have been shown to cause cancer in laboratory animals.

The following are nitrosating agents which can cause nitrosamine contamination:

2-bromo-2-nitropropane-1,3-diol
Ammonium Laureth Sulfate
Ammonium Lauryl Sulfate
Cocoyl Sarcosine
DEA compounds
Formaldehyde
Hydrolysed Animal Protein
Imidazolidinyl Urea
Lauryl Sarcosine
MEA compounds
Quaternium-7, 15, 31, 60, etc.
Sodium Laureth Sulfate
Sodium Lauryl Sulfate
Sodium Methyl Cocoyl Taurate
TEA compounds

Oxybenzone (Benzophenone-3)

Has been shown to cause photoallergic reactions.

 It absorbs through the skin is present in the bodies of 97% of Americans according to the CDC.

Used as a UV blocker in the majority of sunscreens, including children's, lip balms, lip gloss, lipsticks, many lotions and moisturizing creams with SPF listings.
Found in anti-aging creams, shampoo's, conditioners, perfumes, after shave lotions as well as a number of cosmetics products.
Linked to cancer in government, industry and academic studies. Linked to developmental and reproductive toxicity.
Can cause a broad range of health effects from infertility and reproductive organ cancer.
 Birth defects and developmental delays for children. Linked to harm to the immune system, manifest as allergic reactions or impaired capacity to fight desease and repair damaged tissues.

Paraben preservatives (methyl, propyl, butyl, and ethyl)
Used widley as inhibitors of microbial growth to extend shelf life of products even though they are known to be toxic chemicals. Cause many allergic reactions and skin rashes.
Parabens are listed as endocrine disruptors.
Highly toxic chemical.
FROM THE MSDS

WARNING! Harmful if swallowed or inhaled. Causes irritation to skin, eyes and respiratory tract. May cause allergic skin reaction.
SKIN CONTACT: Causes irritation to skin. Symptoms include redness, itching and pain. May cause allergic skin reactions.
EYE CONTACT: Causes irritation, redness and pain.

PCB's

One of the "Dirty Dozen" toxic chemicals banned in April 2001 by the Stockholm Convention.
Japan banned the production, use and import of PCB's in 1972.
The US banned production in 1977 although they are still allowed to be used in closed systems.
The UK banned the use of PCB's in new equipment in 1981 but closed uses were allowed to continue until December 2000.
PCB's continue to this day to enter the enviornment from illegal dumping and disposal of equipment in waste sites and from leaking equipment still allowed to be in use.
PCB's have been linked to cancer, reproductive, neurological and developmental effects and they are endocrine disruptors.

Exposures to infants through breast milk has been linked to lower IQ, hyperactivity, delayed learning, motor skills and short term memory reduction.
Exposures to human, polar bear and whale fetus's have been shown to contribute to reproductive maladies.

In the womb unborn males can be "feminized" or intersex, neither male nor female. Both sets of reproductive organs often develop. PCB's persist in the soil and sediment in water for decades. They accumulate in plant food sources and are their levels increase as they move up the food chain through meat, fish and dairy products. As a result humans, who store them in fatty tissue, can be exposed to levels many times higher than the original concentrations.
 It typically takes 7 to 10 years for the human body to eliminate half of its body burden of these toxic chemicals.

Phthalates
Phthalates are not identified as being present in any of the products which contain them. They are found in products such as IV tubing, vinyl flooring, glues, inks, pesticides, detergents, plastic bags, food packaging.

Its in soaps, shampoos, perfumes, colognes, hair spray, nail polish, vinyl shower curtians, soft plastic children's toys.also infant care products such as powders, lotions and shampoos, many fragrances, adult cosmetics and personal/skin care products.
 Phthalates are not chemically bound to any product so they are continuously being released from the personal care products via skin contact, from vinyl products into the air, leaching into liquids all of which leads to exposure through ingestion, absorption, and inhalation. Animal and human research suggests that early exposure to some phthalates reduces testosterone production.
 And alters the development reproductive organs, particularly in male infants. Some phthalates are known endocrine disruptors.
Common Phthalates are:
butylbenzyl phthalate (BBzP)
di-2-ethylhexyl phthalate (DEHP)
dibutyl phthalate (DBP)
diethyl phthalate (DEP)
di-isononyl phthalate (DiNP)
di-n-octyl phthalate (DnOP)
mono-2-ethyl-5-hydroxyhexyl phthalate (MEHHP)
mono-2-ethyl-5-oxohexyl phthalate (MEOHP)

mono-2-ethylhexyl phthalate (MEHP)
mono-3-carboxypropyl phthalate (MCPP)
monobenzyl phthalate (MBzP)
monoethyl phthalate (MEP)
monoisobutyl phthalate (MiBP)
mono-n-butyl phthalate (MBP)
monomethyl phthalate (MMP)

Polyethylene Glycol (PEG)
A potentially carcinogenic petroleum
ingredient that can alter and reduce the
skin's natural moisture factor.
Used in products designed to dissolve oil
and grease and clean ovens.
Also see
Ethoxylated surfactants

Propylene/Butylene Glycol (PG)
Propylene glycol (PG) is a petroleum by-
product.
It penetrates the skin and can weaken
protein and cellular structure. Commonly
used to make extracts from herbs.

PG penetrates the skin so quickly, the EPA
warns against skin contact to prevent
consequences such as brain, liver, and
kidney abnormalities.

All of this and there isn't even a warning label on products such as stick deodorants, where the concentration is greater than in most industrial applications.
INHALATION: May cause respiratory and throat Irritation, central nervous system depression,
blood and kidney disorders. May cause Nystagmus, Lymphocytosis.
SKIN: Irritation and dermatitis, absorption.
EYES: Irritation and conjunctivitis.
INGESTION: Pulmonary edema, brain damage, hypoglycemia, intravascular hemolysis. Death may occur.

PVP/VA Copolymer
Used in hairsprays, wave sets and some cosmetics.
Particles may contribute to respiratory problems when inhaled into the lungs of sensitive persons.

Quaternium-7, 15, 31, 60, etc.
Prolonged or repeated exposure may cause skin irritation. May cause more severe response if skin is damp. May be a weak skin sensitizer in susceptible individuals at greater than 1% in aqueous solution.
Also see:Nitrosating agents

Rancid Natural Emollients

Rancid natural emollients (oils) form free radicals which damage and age your skin. Natural oils used in cosmetics, such as Borage, Evening Primrose and Rosehip, should be cold pressed not refined.

Creams and lotions made from cold pressed plant oils will have approximately a 6 month use by date.
The reason for this is that they are not refined.
The refining process generates excessive heat which produces "trans" fatty acids some of which are poisonous. The refining process also removes the nutrients, vitamins and essential fatty acids and therefore they contain none of the valuable skin conditioning agents that they were used for in the firsts place.

Silicone derived emollients

Silicone emollients coat the skin and hair trapping anything that is under it. They do not allow the skin or hair to breathe thus leading to skin irritations, acne problems and unhealthy hair.

Some synthetic emollients have been found to cause tumors in laboratory tests and accumulate in the liver and lymph nodes. They are also an environmental concern as they are not biodegradable. Silicone derived emollients include the following:
Cyclomethicone
Dimethicone
Dimethicone Copolyol

Sodium Laureth Sulfate (SLES)
Ammonium Laureth Sulfate (ALES)

When combined with other toxic chemicals, SLES and ALES can create nitrosamines, a potent class of cancer causing carcinogens. They are often hidden in natural and so called organic cosmetics with the words "derived from coconut oil".
FROM THE MSDS WARNING!
Causes skin and eye irritation! Avoid contact with eyes, skin and clothing.
Also see Anionic Surfactants ,Ethoxylated surfactants , Nitrosating agents

Sodium Lauryl Sulfate (SLS) Ammonium Lauryl Sulfate (ALS)

SLS and ALS are found in the vast majority of cosmetics and skin care products that foam. Their primary commercial uses are in car washes, garage floor cleaners and engine degreasers.
Laboratory test show that SLS and ALS cause eye damage, central nervous system depression, labored breathing, diarrhea, severe skin irritation, and even death.
If exposed to SLS and ALS young eyes may not develop properly because proteins are dissolved. SLS and ALS can cause skin layers to separate and inflame.

They are often hidden in so called "natural" and "organic" cosmetics with the words "derived from coconut oil".

Also see Anionic Surfactants , Nitrosating agents

Stearalkonium Chloride

Used in hair conditioners and creams Stearalkonium chloride was originally developed as fabric softener.
It is much less expensive and easier to use than proteins or herbals. Toxic Chemical.
Also see - Cationic surfactants

Talc

Scientific studies have shown that routine application of talcum powder in the genital area is associated with a three-to-fourfold increase in the development of ovarian cancer.

TEA (Triethanolamine) Laureth Sulfate

A highly acidic compound Approximately 40% of cosmetics containing TEA, have been shown to contain nitrosamines, which are potent carcinogens.
FROM THE MSDS Special Hazard Precautions: Product is severely irritating to body tissues and possibly corrosive to the eyes. Handle with care. Avoid eye and skin contact.
Avoid breathing vapors if generated. If there is danger of eye contact, wear a face shield.

Toluene

FROM THE MSDS -POISON! DANGER! Toxic Chemical! Harmful or fatal if swallowed. Harmful if inhaled or absorbed through skin. May affect liver, kidneys, blood system or central nervous system. Causes irritation to skin, eyes and respiratory tract.

INHALATION: Inhalation may cause irritation of the upper respiratory tract. Symptoms of overexposure may include fatigue, confusion, headache, dizziness and drowsiness. Peculiar skin sensations i.e., pins and needles or numbness may be produced. Very high concentrations may cause unconsciousness and death.
INGESTION: Swallowing may cause abdominal spasms and other symptoms that parallel over exposure from inhalation. Aspiration of material into the lungs can cause Chemical Pneumonitis, which may be fatal.
SKIN CONTACT: Causes irritation. May be absorbed through the skin.
EYE CONTACT: Causes severe eye irritation with redness and pain.
CHRONIC EXPOSURE: Reports of chronic poisoning described anemia, decreased blood cell count and bone marrow Hypoplasia. Liver and kidney damage may occur. Repeated or prolonged contact has a defatting action, causing drying, redness and dermatitis.
Exposure of a pregnant woman to toluene may affect a developing fetus.

Toxaphene
One of the "Dirty Dozen" toxic chemicals banned in April 2001 by the Stockholm Convention.

Toxaphene was used as a pesticide replacement for DDT in the mid 1970's. It was banned from general use in the US in 1982 . The US EPA and DHHS have determined the toxaphene is probably a human carcinogen. High levels of exposure can cause damage to lungs, nervous system and kidneys and may also cause death.
Toxaphene persists for many years in soil and sediment in water and is found virtually everywhere in to fresh water and saltwater. It evaporates from the water and travels on air currents. It is most commonly found in certain species of fish. Exposure to humans is most commonly through eating contaminated fish or breathing air near a hazardous waste site. Once consumed by humans it remains stored in fatty tissues for long periods of time. It may be a hazard to the unborn fetus and nursing infants.

If you find any of the toxic chemical ingredients listed here in your cosmetics, skin care products, bath, body and baby products or products you use around you home be sure to get rid of them and replace then with healthy, green natural products.

Final Thought

You arrived here an unknowing participant in the largest human experiment is history.

You have been given very little in the way of good advice and large concerns have lobbied hard and long to keep you confused and part of this ill advised research into just how much we can hurt the body before it kill the whole race.

In every way that matters – you were not to blame.

With that said, if you have read these past pages (and did your homework to be sure I did mine) - you now have no excuse.

You now know why most of what we eat is not human food. You know what human food is. And you have the basic tools to make the right choices.

As with anything, you should move into this with slow and deliberate steps.

Any book like this is really, by design, to simply start you thinking about things in a new light. To help yo move in the right direction.
And for our endeavor, to help you divide the B.S. from the facts.

To challenge the norms is always a scary proposition.

To try and rise above the massive influence that surrounds us - is brave and uncomfortable work.

And to use an over used cliche:
The longest journey begins with a single step.

So, if you take away anything from this – it should be that IT MATTERS!

It matters what you eat, drink and that you are a human – not a test subject. Reject flawed concepts, bad ideas and flat out lies.

With that in mind, here are your 3 tools to bring with you to every choice you make about your health and body.
They appear in the beginning of the book and I leave you with them here at end.

HENDRY'S 3 LAWS FOR HUMANS:

1) Never accept any argument that is made in favor of a chemical and against nature

2) Never accept trading off moments of bliss for years of pain

3) Protect your body and your world – you only get one.

In the end, you are the one that can make the biggest changes in your health.
You have to read.
Fact check.
Stay informed.
And always value your life more than a fad or trend.
Following these simply rules is a huge step on the way to a long and healthy life.

Be well,
RHH

Richard Hendry is a natural health consultant with over 25 years of experience in helping people achieve better health.
Over the past 3 decades he has hosted talk radio shows on natural health, lectured, published natural health magazines, been a contributing writer for newspapers & magazines, promoted Natural health expos and performed over 40,000 natural health screening in 17 states.
He currently lives in Louisville Kentucky where he is a natural health consultant. Richard has also published 25 books of fiction and non-fiction.

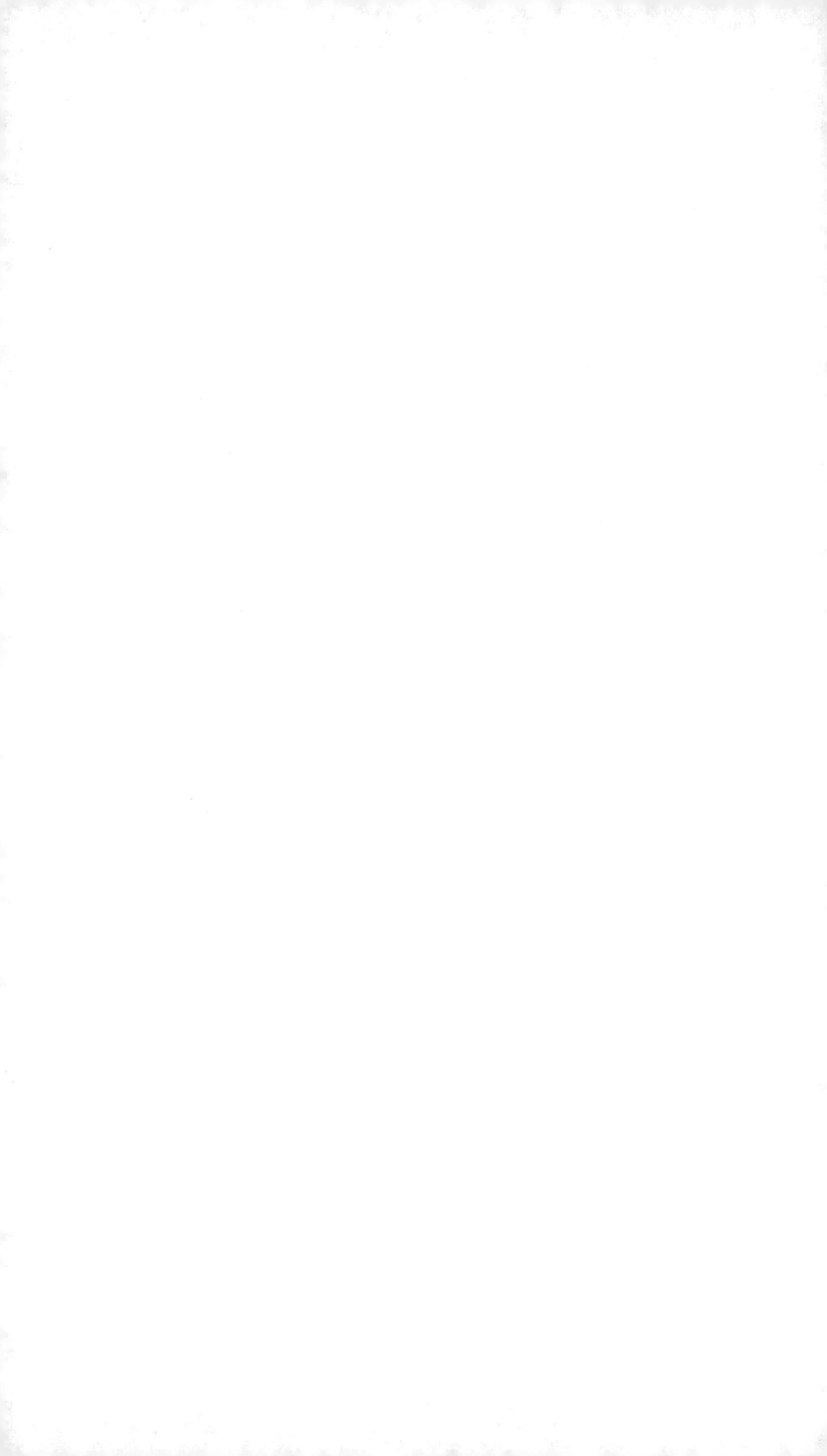

www.ingramcontent.com/pod-product-compliance
Lightning Source LLC
Chambersburg PA
CBHW061806250726
48657CB00001B/317